Sex Drive Smoothie Potion

15 Sensual Smoothies: A Journey to Libido Bliss

Lorrie C. Turner

Copyright/Disclaimer ©

© 2024 Lorrie C. Turner

This book is intended for informational and entertainment purposes only. The information provided in this book is based on the author's personal experiences, research, and knowledge up to the publication date. It is not intended as a substitute for professional medical or nutritional advice.

Readers are advised to consult with healthcare professionals or qualified nutritionists regarding individual health concerns or dietary needs. The author and publisher disclaim any liability arising directly or indirectly from the use of the information provided in this book.

Every effort has been made to ensure that the information in this book is accurate at the time of publication. However, the author and publisher do not assume and hereby disclaim any liability to any party for any loss, damage, or disruption caused by errors or omissions, whether such errors or omissions result from negligence, accident, or any other cause.

Thank you for respecting the intellectual property and legal rights associated with this book.

About the Author: Lorrie C. Turner

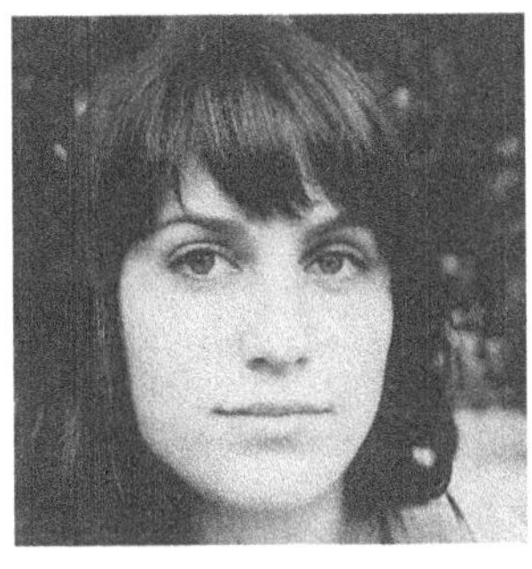 Lorrie C. Turner, a passionate connoisseur of both culinary arts and holistic well-being, brings a unique blend of expertise to the world of sensual smoothies. With a background in nutrition and a flair for crafting delightful elixirs, Lorrie's journey into the intersection of flavors and intimacy has been a labor of love.

As a dedicated enthusiast of creating recipes that not only tantalize the taste buds but also promote overall wellness, Lorrie's exploration of the nexus between nutrition and sensuality is reflected in the carefully curated smoothies presented in this book. With an emphasis on combining exotic ingredients, Lorrie weaves a tapestry of flavors aimed at elevating not just the palate but the intimate experiences of those who embark on this flavorful journey.

Lorrie C. Turner believes in the power of nature's bounty to nourish the body and invigorate the spirit. Her dedication to promoting a holistic approach to pleasure and well-being is evident in the thoughtful selection of ingredients and the expertly crafted recipes within these pages.

Beyond the realm of culinary arts, Lorrie is an advocate for balanced living and strives to inspire others to embrace a lifestyle that harmonizes with the natural rhythms of the body. With a commitment to sharing knowledge and fostering a community of flavor enthusiasts, Lorrie invites readers to join her in this exploration of taste, nutrition, and intimate bliss.

Table of Contents:

Copyright/Disclaimer
About the Author
Introduction
Chapter 1
Link between Nutrition and Libido
    Nutrients Essential for Libido Boosting
    The Role of Antioxidants in Intimacy
    Balancing Macronutrients for Passion
    Superfoods for Sensual Vitality
    Crafting Culinary Aphrodisiacs
Chapter 2
The Art of Crafting Creamy Pleasure Elixirs:
Chapter 3
Recipe 1: Luscious Watermelon and Banana Ecstasy
Chapter 4
Recipe 2: Tropical Tango Passion Blend with Dairy
Chapter 5
Recipe 3: Divine Dark Chocolate Delight
Chapter 6

Recipe 4: Seductive Strawberry Fusion
Chapter 7
Recipe 5: Velvet Vanilla Temptation
Chapter 8
Recipe 6: Mango Bliss Intimacy Infusion
Chapter 9
Recipe 7: Nutty Banana Aphrodisiac Symphony
Chapter 10
Recipe 8: Exotic Pineapple Pleasure Potion
Chapter 11
Recipe 9: Creamy Avocado Velvet Kiss
Chapter 12
Recipe 10: Berry Burst Sensation Elixir
Chapter13
Recipe 11: Citrus Zest Connection Concoction
Chapter 14
Recipe 12: Papaya And Other Tropical Varieties
Chapter 15
Recipe 13: Creamy Fig Fantasy
Chapter 16
Recipe14: Kiwi Kiss Libation

Chapter 17
Recipe 15: Passion Potion
Chapter 18
Conclusion
A Toast to Sensuality and Well-Being
Chapter 19
Review

Introduction

Welcome to "15 Sensual Smoothies: A Journey to Libido Bliss" where enhanced intimacy and delectable nourishment work in perfect harmony. Explore the world of rich drinks made to enhance your sexual pleasure. Learn the techniques behind 15 healthy smoothie recipes that are designed to boost happiness and pleasure for both men and women. Begin your trip toward the pinnacle of sexual ecstasy.

There is a field of uncharted territory at the nexus of sensuality and nutrition, where tastes dance on the tongue and scents conjure up memories in the world of gastronomic joy. Introducing "Sensual Smoothies: A Journey to Libido Bliss," an exclusive collection created to entice your palate and enhance your personal encounters.

Seeking the highest level of enjoyment and well-being has become a necessary endeavor in our hectic lives. Using the abundance of nature, this artwork presents a selection of smoothie recipes that have been painstakingly prepared to not only satisfy your wants but also kindle a passion inside of you. I explore the intriguing area where pleasure and nutrition converge to create elixirs that satiate the body and pique appetites.

Investigating the Nexus of Nutrition and Libido: It is essential to comprehend how nutrition and libido are related. This collection of carefully chosen recipes goes beyond the realm of typical smoothies. Every mixture is an explosion of tastes, textures, and nutrients that have been carefully selected to boost energy, encourage wellness, and reawaken latent desires.

A Harmony of Unusual Ingredients:

As I present to you a symphony of exotic ingredients, from the tempting sweetness of passion fruit to the crispness of apples, the succulence of watermelon, the creaminess of ripe bananas, and the nutty richness of peanuts take a trip through verdant orchids and tropical paradises. Uncovering the secrets these components conceal to enhance your pleasure is the true purpose of this collection.

Making Libido Bliss Elixirs:

Savor the skill of creating elixirs that go beyond the norm. Every dish offers a delicious fusion of tastes that is guaranteed to make you smile. I lead you through the process of creating elixirs that are meant to stimulate desire, arouse blissful passion, and tempt the senses. Some of my favorites include the Luscious Watermelon and Banana Ecstasy, the Tropical Tango Passion Blend with Dairy, and the enticing Passion Potion.

Nourishing the Body and the Soul:
Going Beyond Taste
These smoothies are meant to feed the body and the spirit, not simply the palate. I explore the functions of antioxidants, macronutrients, and particular foods known for their aphrodisiac properties as I dig into the dietary components that support general well-being. Let every sip serve as a springboard for a more flavorful and full life as well as a healthy one.

Chapter 1

Link between Nutrition and Libido

There is a strong correlation between diet and libido. Foods high in nutrients promote blood flow, hormone production, and general health—all important components of a strong sex drive.

Nutrition's relationship to The science of libido explains how certain vitamins, minerals, and antioxidants enhance intimate vitality and provide the groundwork for a happy and pleasurable sexual encounter.

• Nutrients Essential for Sex Drive/Libido Boosting:

Examining the particular nutrients that are essential for maintaining hormone balance, blood flow, and general sexual health will help us better understand the complex link between diet and desire. We explore the vital vitamins and minerals that support a strong and active sex drive in this section.

1. Zinc:

Function: Essential for the synthesis of testosterone, the main sex hormone in men.

Fruit Sources: Guava, blackberries, kiwi, raspberries, apricots

Other Food Sources:Lentils, beef, oysters, and pumpkin seeds.

2. Vitamin (D)

Function: Associated with testosterone levels and essential for reproductive health in general.

Sources: fortified dairy products and cereals, and fatty fish (salmon, mackerel, tuna), Sunlight.

3. B-Complex Vitamin:
Function: B vitamins, particularly B6, B9 (folate), and B12, aid in the synthesis of red blood cells and the control of hormones.

Fruit Sources: Avocado (B5, B6), banana (B6), citrus fruits (B1, B2, B3, B5, B6), berries (B1, B2, B3, B5, B6), melons (B1, B3, B6), mango (B6), watermelon (B1, B6), papaya (B9)

Additional Food Sources: Nuts, meat, dairy, eggs, whole grains, and leafy greens.

4. Magnesium
Function: Promotes calmness and lowers tension by assisting with muscular function and relaxation.

Fruit Sources: Bananas, avocados, figs, kiwi, papaya, guava, mangoes, blackberries, oranges, strawberries.

Other Food Sources: Leafy greens, legumes, nuts, and seeds.

5. Iron:

Function: Crucial to the synthesis of hemoglobin, which enhances oxygenation and blood flow.

Fruit Sources: Apricots, prunes, raisins, watermelon, peaches, mulberries, dates, blackcurrants, strawberries.

Other Food Sources: Fish, chicken, lentils, spinach, red meat, and other foods.

6. Fatty Acids Omega-3:

Function: Assist with better blood circulation and cardiovascular health.

Fruit Sources: Chia seeds, flaxseeds, walnuts, hemp seeds, kiwi seeds, raspberries, blackberries, strawberries, blueberries, mangoes.

Additional Food Sources: walnuts, chia seeds, flaxseeds, and fatty fish (trout, salmon).

7. Vitamin C:
Function: Promotes blood circulation and aids in the production of hormones such as estrogen.

Fruit Sources: Berries, citrus fruits, kiwi, pineapple, mango, guava, papaya, cantaloupe, watermelon.
Other Food Sources: Broccoli, bell peppers.

8. Vitamin E
Function: Serves as an antioxidant to safeguard cells and maintain hormonal equilibrium.
Fruit Sources: All berries, kiwi, mango, avocado, papaya, apricots.
Other food sources include nuts, seeds, spinach, broccoli, and sunflower oil.

9. Selenium:

Function: Contributes to the synthesis of sperm and testosterone.

Fruit Sources: Bananas, oranges, strawberries, grapes, watermelon.

Other Food Sources: Whole grains, fish, chicken, and brazil nuts.

10. L-Arginine

Function: Amino acid that promotes blood flow by assisting in the synthesis of nitric oxide.

Fruit Sources: watermelon, pineapple, grapes, kiwi, guava, mango, papaya, blackberries, strawberries, avocado.

Additional Food Sources: Dairy, almonds, seeds, poultry, and red meat.

These nutrient-dense foods provide the groundwork for hormonal balance and healthy sexual function when you include them in your diet. Remember that a healthy lifestyle and a diverse, balanced food improve general well-being, which in turn boosts libido in both men and women.

These vital nutrients are more than just food; they are the cornerstone of a more fulfilling and healthful personal life.

• The Role of Antioxidants in Intimacy

Strong protectors against oxidative stress and cellular damage, antioxidants are essential for interpersonal well-being. Their impact on
sexuality includes blood flow enhancement, cardiovascular health support, and reproductive cell protection.
 Let us investigate the role that antioxidants play in the complex dance of intimacy.

☐ Enhanced Blood Circulation: Antioxidants help to increase blood circulation by scavenging free radicals. Increased blood flow is essential for sexual function because it makes sure that the reproductive organs get oxygen and nutrients in an effective manner. A better sexual response and higher level of excitement may result from this enhanced circulation.

- ☐ Cardiovascular Support: For personal well-being, the cardiovascular system's health is crucial. Antioxidants support cardiovascular health by lowering inflammation and avoiding oxidative blood vessel damage. Overall sexual function is supported by a healthy heart, which guarantees appropriate blood flow to all body areas, including the genital area.

- ☐ Preserving Reproductive Cells: Sperm quality and egg health may be negatively impacted by oxidative stress, which can affect reproductive cells. Antioxidants function as barriers, preventing harm to these cells and preserving the integrity of the reproductive system. This may improve the viability and motility of sperm in males, and it can help women produce better eggs.

☐ Stress Reduction: Chronic stress, which may have a detrimental effect on libido, is directly associated with oxidative stress. Antioxidants aid in reducing stress by reducing oxidative stress. A more at ease mental state creates an atmosphere that is favorable for closeness and enhances the quality of the sexual encounter.

☐ Hormonal Balance: Antioxidants influence the synthesis and control of many hormones linked to sexual function, helping to maintain hormonal balance. For both men and women, maintaining this balance is essential to a healthy libido and general sexual well-being.

☐ Enhanced Sexual Response: Antioxidants assist hormonal balance, better blood flow, and cardiovascular support, all of which add to an enhanced sexual response. A more satisfying intimate encounter may result from heightened sensitivity, arousal, and contentment in a couple.

Excellent Fruit Sources Of Antioxidants:
- Berries: Cranberries, blackberries, strawberries, raspberries, and blueberries
- Citrus Fruits: grapefruit, oranges, limes, tangerine and lemons.
- Tropical fruits: guavas, papayas, pineapples, and mangoes.
- Stone Fruits: Apricots, plums, peaches, and cherries.
- Pears and Apples
- Grapes: Black and red grapes
- Kiwi: Gold and green varieties
- Avocado - Tomatoes - Watermelon

NOTE: Including a range of these fruits, which are high in antioxidants, in your smoothies may improve your general health and well-being. This includes possible advantages for intimacy as well as support for cardiovascular health.

Furthermore, adopting a lifestyle that prioritizes stress reduction, regular exercise, and a balanced diet enhances the beneficial effects of antioxidants on intimate health.

• Balancing Macronutrients for Passion

A well-balanced diet with the correct ratio of macronutrients is essential for pursuing passions. In this article, we explore the importance of every macronutrient and how maintaining their proper balance promotes a life filled with passion and energy.

1. Carbohydrates

- Function: The body uses carbohydrates as its main energy source. Energy levels must be maintained and physical activity must be fueled by carbohydrates.

- Passionate Link: An energy source that never runs out guarantees endurance and stamina, which helps maintain desire during intimate times.

- Fruit sources include bananas, apples, kiwis, mangoes, pineapples, oranges, berries, and grapes.

2. Proteins

- Function: Components that make up tissues, such as muscles and hormones. Proteins aid in the synthesis of vital hormones and enzymes as well as muscle development and repair.

- Passion Connection: Consuming enough protein builds muscular strength and endurance, which are necessary for engaging in physically demanding activities.

- Fruit Sources: Oranges, bananas, peaches, passion fruits, guavas, avocados, apricots, and kiwis

3. Fats.
   - Function: Critical for the synthesis of hormones and the uptake of fat-soluble vitamins. Heart health is one aspect of general well-being that is enhanced by healthy fats.
   - Passion Connection: Heart health, which is essential for proper blood flow and personal well-being, is supported by fats, especially omega-3 fatty acids.
   Fruit Sources: hemp seeds, walnuts, flaxseeds, and chia seeds.

4. Complex vs. Simple Carbohydrates
   - Function: Complex carbohydrates provide you long-lasting energy, whilst simple carbs give you short spurts.
   - Passion Connection: Selecting complex carbs during times of passion gives you a

more consistent and long-lasting energy source.

☐ Complex Carbohydrates:
Fruit sources include pears, apples, berries, grapes and oranges.

☐ Simple carbohydrates:
Fruit Sources: Watermelon, papayas, mangoes, pineapples, bananas, etc.
Additional Sources: legumes, whole grains, etc.

5. Healthy Fats versus Lean Fats

- Function: Healthy fats and lean proteins promote general health without causing overconsumption of calories.

- Passion Connection: Including heart-healthy fats in your diet, including those in nuts and avocados, and selecting lean protein sources are key components of a balanced, heart-healthy diet.

6. Macronutrient Ratio Balancing

- Function: Maintaining a healthy balance of macronutrients is essential for energy balance and general health.

- Passionate Connection ; The body receives the resources it needs to perform at its best from a well-balanced diet, which supports passion's emotional and physical dimensions.

7. water

- Function: Although not a macronutrient, enough water is necessary for digestion, nutrition transfer, and general health.

- Passion Connection: Maintaining proper hydration during passionate times is essential for sustaining energy levels and supporting body functions.

- Gut Health and Libido Connection

Often called the "second brain," the stomach is essential to general health and has an impact on personal well-being as well.

☐ Microbiome and Hormonal Balance

- Role: Hormone control, particularly that of sexually active hormones like testosterone and estrogen, is influenced by the gut microbiota.

- Libido Connection: Harmonious hormone levels, which maintain a healthy libido in both men and women, are facilitated by a balanced microbiota.

☐ Production of Serotonin

- Role: The stomach produces a large quantity of serotonin, a neurotransmitter linked to mood and wellbeing.

- Libido Connection: Elevated serotonin levels promote a cheerful disposition, lessen stress and anxiety, and create an atmosphere that is favorable for closeness.

☐ Nutrient Absorption

- Role: The intestines play a major role in the absorption of vital nutrients, including zinc and vitamin D, which are important for sexual health.

- Libido Connection: Nutrient absorption that promotes libido and general intimate well-being is made possible by a gut that is operating at optimal capacity.

☐ Probiotics and Libido
- Function: Probiotics, which are good bacteria present in certain foods and supplements including kimchi, pickles, and yogurt, help maintain a balanced population of gut flora.

- Libido Connection: Probiotics may help maintain a healthy and diversified microbiome, which can have a good effect on sexual function and libido.

☐ Libido and Inflammation
- Role: Inflammation is a result of gut dysbiosis and may have a detrimental impact on general health, including sexual function.
- Libido Connection: An atmosphere that promotes good intimate well-being is

fostered by decreased inflammation, which is a result of a healthy gut.

□ Stress Response
- Role: The body's reaction to stress is influenced by the gut-brain axis, which is the two-way communication between the gut and the brain.
- Libido Connection: Having a healthy gut makes one more robust to stress, which enhances libido and enhances sexual pleasure.

□ Fiber and Gut Health
- Function: Dietary fiber, which is included in fruits and vegetables including apples, bananas, oranges, berries, spinach, avocados, mangos, and whole grains, plays a role in supporting gut health by encouraging the development of good bacteria.
- The Libido Connection: Eating a high-fiber diet helps maintain a healthy gut, which in turn supports libido by sustaining general wellbeing.

• **Superfoods for Sensual Vitality**

When it comes to achieving sensuous vitality, several "superfoods" are particularly effective at promoting general health, which includes sexual wellness.

1. Dark Chocolate

It has aphrodisiac properties because it produces endorphins, which provide pleasure, and contains chemicals like phenylethylamine, which is linked to feelings of love.

Nutrient Boost: Packed with antioxidants, which support healthy cardiovascular function and blood flow.

2. Avocado

Velvety Texture: Avocados' rich, creamy texture may give dishes a posh touch and a sensuous feel.

Rich in potassium, vitamin E, and heart-healthy fats, this nutrient profile supports cardiovascular health.

3. Strawberries

Sensuous Symbol: Packed in antioxidants and vitamin C, strawberries may be fed to others and shared in a sensuous way.

Nutrient Profile: Contains chemicals linked to increased sensitivity and improves blood flow.

4. Nuts (peanuts, walnuts, and almonds):

Crunchy Pleasure: Nuts give food a gratifying crunch and give meals and snacks texture.

Nutrient Boost: Packed with zinc, vitamin E, and healthy fats that promote hormone synthesis and cardiovascular health.

5. Pomegranate

Juicy Delight: Pomegranates' vivid, juicy seeds may improve a dish's aesthetic appeal.

Rich in antioxidants, this nutrient profile may help with erectile dysfunction and heart health.

6. Watermelon:

Hydrating Refreshment: Watermelon's high water content may provide for a hydrating and refreshing experience.

Nutrient Profile: Citrulline is present and may be advantageous for intimate health and blood flow.

7. Figs:

Sweet Treat: Figs lend a delicious sweetness to savory and sweet meals since they are inherently sweet.

Nutrient Boost: Rich in fiber, which supports healthy digestion; also contains magnesium and manganese.

7. Chia Seeds:

Texture Enhancement: When soaked, chia seeds take on a gelatinous texture that gives food a special touch.

Nutrient Profile: High in fiber, protein, and omega-3 fatty acids, which promote general well being.

• Crafting Culinary Aphrodisiacs

This is the art of putting your heart and soul into your cooking, with an emphasis on employing natural aphrodisiacs. This delves into the sensuous realm of tastes, textures, and fragrances that may enhance your meals and make dining with your partner a special and enjoyable experience.

1. Vanilla

Aromatic Elegance: Vanilla's warm, sweet aroma may evoke a passionate mood.

Culinary Use: A hint of vanilla may improve drinks, sweets, and even savory foods.

2. Cinnamon

Spicy Warmth: Due to its warming qualities, cinnamon gives food a hint of spice.

Culinary Use: For a tasty touch, add to smoothies, desserts, or drinks as a sprinkle or infusion.

3. Honey

Sweet Indulgence: Honey's inherent sweetness gives food a sumptuous touch.

Culinary Use: Use as a natural sweetener in a variety of dishes, or drizzle over fruits or blend into yogurt.

4. Ginseng

Energizing elixir: It is said that ginseng has stimulating qualities that encourage vigor and energy.

Culinary Use: For a mild flavor boost, infuse into teas, blend into soups, or use in stir-fries.

5. Saffron

Exotic Elegance: The distinct taste and vivid color of saffron may raise food to a whole new level.

Culinary Use: For a sophisticated touch, add a pinch to rice, soups, or desserts.

6. Basil

Herbal Sensation: The fragrant and fresh taste characteristic of basil gives food a flavor boost.

Culinary Use: Incorporate into salads, sauces, or as a garnish to provide a touch of herbal flavor.

7. Olive Oil

Liquid Gold: Rich and smooth mouthfeel is a result of using premium olive oil.

Culinary Use: Use as a dip, drizzle over salads, or infuse with herbs to create a flavorful infusion that is sensuous.

8. Cardamom

Exotic Spice: The somewhat sweet and fragrant flavor of cardamom lends an air of exoticism.

Culinary Use: Add to coffee, sweets, or even savory foods to create a fragrant and distinct flavor.

9. Rosemary

Herbal Elegance: A range of foods may benefit from the fragrant, pine-like taste of rosemary.

Culinary Use: Incorporate into oils, marinades, or roasted meats for a flavorful culinary experience.

10. Chocolate
Rich and smooth, chocolate satisfies all the senses. Decadent Delight.

Culinary Use: Add to drinks, sweets, or even savory meals for a tasty treat.

Chapter 2

The Art of Crafting Creamy Pleasure Elixirs:

This combination of tastes, textures, and sustaining ingredients results in creamy elixirs that are more than just drinks; they're declarations of love and passion. This part reveals the techniques for creating silky mixtures that enhance the personal experience while also pleasing the palate.

1. **Velvety Bases**

Sensual feel: Start with a foundation that gives your elixir a rich, velvety feel.

Almond milk, Greek yogurt, and coconut milk are a few examples.

2. **A Harmony of Tastes**

Balanced Harmony: To produce a well-rounded and alluring character, combine a range of tastes.

Examples include nutmeg, cinnamon, honey, and vanilla.

3. **Aphrodisiacal Infusions**

Passionate Boost: Incorporate natural aphrodisiacs into your elixir to arouse desire.

Avocado, strawberries, and dark chocolate are a few examples.

4. **Supplements Rich in Nutrients**

Vitality Infusion: Combine components that are high in vital nutrients to promote general health.

Examples include spinach, flaxseeds, and chia seeds.

5. **Sweet Serenades**

Natural Sweeteners: Choose sweeteners that subtly enhance the elixir's sweetness.

Dates, maple syrup, and agave nectar are a few examples.

6. Tropical Temptations

Exotic Allure: To give a fascinating and exotic touch, include tropical fruits.

Mango, pineapple, and passion fruit are among examples.

7. Nutty Nuances

Creamy Depth: Add nuts to create a deep, nutty flavor.

Walnuts, cashew nuts, groundnuts, and almonds are a few examples.

8. Superfoods for Smoothies

Energizing Elements: Upgrade your concoction with superfoods renowned for their superior nutritional value.

Spirulina, maca powder, and acai berries are a few examples.

9. Temperature Play

Hot or Cold: Take into account the occasion and your own tastes while choosing the temperature of your elixir.

Examples: Ice for a cool twist or warm spices for a comforting elixir.

10. **Use a graceful garnish**

Visual Appeal: Use tasteful garnishes to give a touch of elegance and elevate the presentation.

Examples include grated dark chocolate, edible flowers, and mint leaves.

Making creamy pleasure elixirs is a personal art form that involves more than just putting ingredients together.

**NOTE: These Recipes
are made for two or
more people.**

**It should be taken just
before having sex
with your partner.**

**And better results are
achieved when taken
together with your
sex partner.**

Chapter 3

Recipe 1: Luscious Watermelon and Banana Ecstasy

Four Ingredients Needed:

- 3 cups fresh watermelon, diced
- 3 ripe bananas, sliced
- 4 tablespoons peanut butter
- 2 cup Greek yogurt
- Ice cubes (optional)

Instructions:

1. Gather the Ingredients:
   - Peel and cut up a fresh watermelon (discard the back).

- Slice the banana after removing the skins.
 - Assemble the remaining components for convenient use.

2. Chill the Ingredients:
 - Refrigerate the bananas and watermelon cubes for 30 minutes, or add ice cubes; alternatively, chill the smoothie after mixing for an even more delightful experience.

3. Blending Magic:
 - Place the Greek yogurt, watermelon, and banana in a blender. Blend until a rough consistency is achieved, then add the peanut butter and ice cubes to the puree. Blend until creamy and smooth, being sure to fully integrate all of the ingredients.

4. Serve in Style:
 - Transfer the decadent concoction into glasses of your choosing.

Chapter 4

Recipe 2: Tropical Tango Passion Blend with Dairy

Six Ingredients needed:

- 3 ripe bananas
- 1 cup Greek yogurt
- 1 cup coconut milk or 1 cup whole coconut, diced.
- 3 tablespoons peanut butter
- ½ cup vodka
- Ice cubes
- Orange slices for garnish (optional)

Instructions:

1. Gather the ingredients:
    - Peel and slice the banana in half lengthwise.

- Collect ice cubes, vodka, coconut milk, and Greek yogurt.

2. Blending Brilliance:
   - Place the banana in a blender together with the Greek yogurt, peanut butter and coconut milk, add the vodka and a few ice cubes.
   - Process the ingredients until it has a creamy, smooth consistency.

3. Present in Style:
   - Transfer the tropical mixture into glasses of your choice.
   - Cool to the appropriate temperature.
   - If orange slices are available, garnish with them.

Chapter 5

Recipe 3: Divine Dark Chocolate Delight

Seven Ingredients Needed:

- 2 cups almond milk
- ½ cup dark chocolate chips (70% cocoa or higher)
- 2 tablespoons unsweetened cocoa powder
- 2 tablespoons honey or any sweetener of choice (adjust to taste)
- ½ teaspoon vanilla extract
- ½ cup Greek yogurt
- 1 ripe banana, sliced for garnish
- Whipped cream for garnish (optional)

Instructions:

1. Gather the ingredients:

- Measure the Greek yogurt, whipped cream, dark chocolate shavings, almond milk, dark chocolate chips, unsweetened cocoa powder, honey, and vanilla essence.
- Peel and slice the banana.

2. Melt the Dark Chocolate:
- Place the dark chocolate chips in a saucepan and heat over low heat, stirring regularly, until the chocolate is smooth.
- Take care not to overheat; when completely melted, remove from heat.

3. Blend the Chocolate Base:
- Put melted dark chocolate, almond milk, cocoa powder, honey and vanilla essence, into a blender.
- Blend until fully incorporated and the mixture is smooth.

4. Cool and Chill:
- To bring out the richness of the elixir, let the chocolate mixture settle to room

temperature and then chill it in the refrigerator for at least 45 minutes.

5. Assemble the Elixir:
   - After the chocolate mix has cooled, transfer it into glasses, making sure there is room for the layers.
   - Place a layer of Greek yogurt in each glass on top of the chocolate mixture.

6. Banana Bliss:
   - To create a delicious fruity accent, place banana slices on top of the Greek yogurt layer.

7. Add Whipped Cream as a Garnish: Drizzle a generous amount of whipped cream into each glass, covering the banana slices in a layer resembling clouds.

9. Present this Divine Dark Chocolate Delight in tall glasses to highlight the layers of decadence and serve with style.

Chapter 6

Recipe 4: Seductive Strawberry Fusion

Five Ingredients Needed:

- 1 cup fresh strawberries, hulled
- ½ cup plain yogurt
- 1 cup coconut milk
- 2 tablespoon honey (adjust to taste)
- Ice cubes

Instructions:

1. Get the strawberries ready:
   - Slice fresh strawberries to make mixing easier after hulling them and removing the green tips.

2. Blending Brilliance:

- Place together the fresh strawberries, plain yogurt, honey, and coconut milk in a blender. Blend till creamy and smooth.

4. Chill and Serve:
   - To improve the taste and coolness, place the Seductive Strawberry Fusion in the refrigerator for half an hour.
   - Ladle the cooled concoction into glasses with ice cubes under.

Chapter 7

Recipe 5: Velvet Vanilla Temptation

Seven Ingredients Needed:

- 2 cups almond milk
- 1 tablespoon vanilla extract
- 2 tablespoons honey (adjust to taste)
- ¼ cup heavy cream
- ¼ cup Greek yogurt
- Ice cubes
- Ground cinnamon for garnish (optional)

Instructions:

1. Blend the Vanilla Base:

- Put the almond milk, honey, vanilla extract, Greek yogurt and heavy cream, in a blender.
- Blend to incorporate and get a smooth, frothy mixture.

2. Chill and Serve:
- To improve the creaminess and chill factor, place the Velvet Vanilla Temptation in the refrigerator for a minimum of half an hour.
- Over ice cubes, pour the cooled elixir into glasses.

4. Sprinkle Cinnamon Magic:
- To create a cozy and welcoming scent, lightly dust each glass with a little ground cinnamon.

Chapter 8

Recipe 6: Mango Bliss Intimacy Infusion

Eight Ingredients Needed:

- 2 cups ripe mango, peeled and diced
- 1 ripe banana
- 1 cup coconut water
- ½ cup plain yogurt
- 2 tablespoons honey (adjust to taste)
 - 3 tablespoons peanut butter
- 1 tablespoon lime juice
- Ice cubes
- Fresh basil leaves for garnish (optional)

Instructions:

1. Preparations:
   - First, make sure the mangoes are ripe for optimum sweetness; then peel and dice them.
   - Peel and slice the banana.

2. Blending Brilliance:
   - Put the banana, peanut butter, plain yogurt, honey, lime juice, and sliced ripe mango in a blender. Blend the ingredients until it becomes silky and luxurious.

3. Chill and Serve:
   - To improve the chill and accentuate the flavors, refrigerate the mango elixir for a minimum of forty minutes.
   - Over ice cubes, pour the cooled elixir into glasses.

4. Garnish with Basil Elegance:

- To add an aromatic touch and a touch of style, garnish each glass with fresh basil leaves, if available.

Chapter 9

Recipe 7: Nutty Banana Aphrodisiac Symphony

Seven Ingredients Needed:

- 3 ripe bananas
- 2 cups almond milk
- ¼ cup almond butter
- ½ teaspoon vanilla extract
- ¼ teaspoon cinnamon
- Ice cubes
- Crushed almonds for garnish

Instruction:

1. Ready the Bananas:
    - Cut and peel ripe bananas to make mixing easier.

2. Blending Brilliance:
   - Place the sliced ripe bananas, almond butter, almond milk, cinnamon and vanilla essence in a blender.
   - Process the ingredients until it has a creamy, smooth consistency.

4. cold and Serve:
   - To increase the cool and deepen the flavors, place the Nutty Banana Aphrodisiac Symphony in the refrigerator for at least one hour.
  - Over ice cubes, pour the chilled elixir into glasses.

5. Add a Nutty Crunch Garnish:
   - Top each glass with a dusting of crushed almonds for a wonderful crunch and aesthetic appeal.

Chapter 10

Recipe 8: Exotic Pineapple Pleasure Potion

Five Ingredients Needed:

- 2 cups fresh pineapple chunks
- 1 cup coconut milk
- ½ cup plain yogurt
- 1 ripe banana
- 1 tablespoons honey (optional)
- Ice cubes

Instructions:

1. Preparations:
   - First, make sure the pineapple is ripe for the best sweetness; then cut it into bits.

- Peel and slice the banana.

2. Blending Brilliance:
   - Put the sliced fresh pineapple, coconut milk, plain yogurt, honey, and banana pieces in a blender. Blend the ingredients until it's smooth and tastes like a tropical paradise.

4. Chill and Serve: - To increase the chill and heighten the tropical tastes, refrigerate the Pineapple Pleasure Potion for at least one hour.
   - Over ice cubes, pour the cooled elixir into glasses.

Chapter 11

Recipe 9: Creamy Avocado Velvet Kiss

Seven Ingredients Needed:

- 2 ripe avocados, peeled and pitted
- 1 cup almond milk
- 1 cup coconut milk
- ¼ cup honey or maple syrup (adjust to taste)
- 1 teaspoon vanilla extract
- 2 tablespoons almond powder or flakes (garnish)
- Ice cubes
- 3 fresh lettuce or spinach (optional)

Instructions:

1. Prepare the Avocados:
   - Peel and pit the ripe avocados, ensuring they are soft and ready for blending.

2. Blending Brilliance:
   - In a blender, combine the ripe avocados, almond milk, coconut milk, honey, vanilla extract and lettuce or spinach.
   - Blend until the mixture is smooth and achieves a velvety consistency.

4. Chill and Serve:
   - Refrigerate the Avocado Velvet Kiss for at least 45 minutes to enhance the chill and creaminess.
   - Pour the chilled elixir into glasses over ice cubes.

5. Garnish with Elegance:
   - Garnish with flaked or powdered almonds.

Chapter 12

Recipe 10: Berry Burst Sensation Elixir

Five Ingredients Needed:

- 2 cups mixed berries (strawberries, blueberries, raspberries)
- 1 cup cranberry juice
- 1 cup plain yogurt
- 1 tablespoon lime juice
- Fresh mint leaves for garnish (optional)
- Ice cubes

Instructions:

1. Get the Berries Ready:
   - Clean and seed strawberries. Make sure the raspberries and blueberries are washed and prepared for mixing.

2. Blending Brilliance:
  - Put the plain yogurt, lime juice, cranberry juice, and mixed berries in a blender. Blend until smooth and the colorful essence of the many berries is captured in the concoction.

4. Chill and Serve:
  - To improve the coolness and heighten the berry tastes, refrigerate the Berry Burst Sensation Elixir for a minimum of 40 minutes.
  - Over ice cubes, pour the cooled elixir into glasses.

5. Garnish with Mint Freshness:
  - For a scent and mental lift, garnish each glass with fresh mint leaves, if available.

Chapter 13

Recipe 11: Citrus Zest Connection Concoction

Six Ingredients Needed:

- 2 sweet oranges, peeled and segmented
- 1 cup grapes or 10 pieces
- 1 lemon, juiced
- 2 cups of milk (full cream)
- Fresh mint leaves for garnish
- Ice cubes

Instructions:

1. Preparation:

- First, make sure the oranges are seed-free by peeling and segmenting them.
  - Clean the grapes.

2. Citrus Juicing Brilliance:
   - Squeeze the lemon to extract its juice, either by hand or in a juicer.

3. Blending the Citrus Symphony:
  - Place the orange segments, grapes, milk, and lemon juice in a blender.
  - Blend until the mixture is well blended and embodies the zesty flavor of citrus blended with dairy.

5. Chill and Serve:

   - To increase the coolness and heighten the citrus tastes, refrigerate the Citrus Zest Connection Concoction for at least one hour.
   - Transfer the cold mixture into glasses with ice cubes on top.

6. If mint freshness is available, garnish.

Chapter 14

Recipe 12: Papaya And Other Tropical Varieties

Six Ingredients Needed:

- 1 cup pineapple chunks
- ½ cup mango chunks
- 2 cups papaya chunks
- ½ cup coconut milk
- ½ cup milk of choice
- Ice cubes

Instructions:

1. Preparation:

- Get the tropical fruits ready. Chop the papaya, mango, and pineapple into large pieces. Make sure the fruits are fully ripe for maximum sweetness.

2. Blending the Tropical Tango:
   - Put the pineapple, mango, and papaya pieces, coconut milk, and milk in a blender. Blend the ingredients until it's smooth and has a hint of tropical flavor.

4. Chill and Serve:
   - To improve the coolness and heighten the tropical flavors, refrigerate the Tropical Tango Passion Blend for a minimum of one hour.
   - Transfer the cool mixture into glasses with ice cubes inside.

Chapter 15

Recipe 13: Creamy Fig Fantasy

Seven Ingredients Needed:

- 2 cups fresh figs, stems removed and halved
- 1 cup Greek yogurt
- ½ cup almond or soy milk
- 2 tablespoons honey (adjust to taste)
- 1 teaspoon vanilla extract
- A pinch of cinnamon
- Ice cubes
-Chopped pistachios for garnish (optional)

Instructions:

1. Ready the Figs:

- Cut the stems off of fresh figs and cut them in half so that blending will be simple.

2. Blending Brilliance:
   - Put the fresh figs, Greek yogurt, sugar, almond or soy milk, vanilla essence, and a dash of cinnamon in a blender. Blend until the mixture is silky smooth and fig essence is captured.

4. Chill and Serve:
 - To increase the coolness and accentuate the fig tastes, place the Creamy Fig Fantasy in the refrigerator for at least 45 minutes.
   - Over ice cubes, pour the cooled elixir into glasses.

5. Add a Pistachio Elegance Garnish: If available, top each glass with chopped pistachios for a wonderful crunch and aesthetic appeal.

Chapter 16

Recipe14: Kiwi Kiss Libation

Five Ingredients Needed:

- 4 ripe kiwis, peeled and sliced
- 1 cup pineapple chunks
- 2 Tablespoons maple syrup
- 1 cup coconut milk
- Ice cubes

Instructions:

1. Preparation:
   - To make mixing easier, peel and slice ripe kiwis.
   - Peel and slice the pineapple.

2. Blending Brilliance:

- Put the chopped pineapple, sliced kiwis, maple syrup, and coconut milk in a blender. Process until the mixture is smooth and has a hint of kiwi flavor.

4. Chill and Serve:
- To improve the chill and accentuate the kiwi tastes, place the Kiwi Kiss Libation in the refrigerator for at least one hour.
- Transfer the cooled concoction into glasses with ice cubes on top.

Chapter 17

Recipe 15: Passion Potion.

Six Ingredients Needed:

- 1 passion fruit pulp (strained)
- 2 apples (cored and sliced)
- 2 cups watermelon (peeled and cubed)
- 1 ripe banana
- 1 cup soy milk
- 3 tablespoons peanut butter

Instructions:

1. Prepare the Ingredients:
   - Using a sieve, remove the juice and pulp from the passion fruit.
   - Cut the apples into thin slices.
   - Peel and slice the watermelon.
   - Peel and slice the ripe banana.

2. Blending Brilliance:
 - Put the watermelon, ripe banana, apples, passion fruit juice, and soy milk in a blender.
    - Process the ingredients until it has a creamy, smooth consistency.

3. Add Nutty Goodness:
    - Place the peanut in the blender and process just long enough to leave tiny, textural pieces of nutty goodness.

4. Verify Consistency:
    - Verify the smoothie's consistency. Increase the soy milk if it's too thick, and increase the fruit or ice cubes if it's too thin.

5. Chill and Serve:
   - To improve the chill, place the Passion Potion in the refrigerator for at least half an hour.
 - Fill glasses with the chilled smoothie.

6. Garnish (Optional):

To add a little more visual appeal, top with a sprinkling of groundnuts or a piece of watermelon.

Conclusion

A Toast to Sensuality and Well-Being

As we reach the final pages of "Sensual Smoothies: A Journey to Libido Bliss," it is with a heartfelt sense of fulfillment and anticipation that I invite you to savor this concluding moment. This piece of art has been a labor of love, an exploration into the realms of taste, desire, and holistic well-being, and it is my sincere hope that it has ignited a flame of passion within you.

Throughout these pages, we have ventured beyond the boundaries of conventional smoothie recipes. We embarked on a journey where nutrition meets sensuality.

Our exploration extended beyond the flavors, delving into the nutritional elements that contribute to overall well-being. The connection between nutrition and libido is a theme that underscores the importance of embracing a holistic approach to pleasure and health. Each ingredient, carefully selected and blended, is an invitation to nourish both the body and the soul.

As you close the cover of this book, I encourage you to carry these recipes into your daily life. Let them be a source of inspiration, a catalyst for crafting moments of bliss, and a reminder that pleasure and wellness are intertwined. Share these elixirs with loved ones, create moments of intimacy, and celebrate the sensory experience of each flavorful sip.

May "Sensual Smoothies" be more than a collection of recipes; may it be a companion on your journey towards a life filled with indulgent moments and heightened satisfaction. May the flavors linger on your palate, and the nutritional wisdom resonate within, guiding you towards a path of holistic well-being.

Here's to your continued exploration of taste, desire, and the vibrant tapestry of life. May every sip be a toast to sensuality and well-being.

With gratitude and wishes for a flavorful and fulfilling journey,

Review

Dear Readers,

If you've had the pleasure of experiencing "Sensual Smoothies: A Journey to Libido Bliss," I would be immensely grateful for your insights. Your thoughts are invaluable in shaping the narrative of this flavorful journey. Could you kindly share your review, detailing your favorite recipes, the impact they had on your sensory experiences, and how the book contributed to your understanding of the connection between nutrition and sensuality? Your feedback will not only aid in refining future editions but will also inspire others to embark on this delicious and holistic exploration.

Thank you for taking the time to share your thoughts!

Warm Regards,
Lorrie C. Turner

www.ingramcontent.com/pod-product-compliance
Lightning Source LLC
Chambersburg PA
CBHW050840260726
48660CB00006B/2355